He

MW01533140

The Complete Guide On How To Treat Bowel Polyps Using Herbs

Dr. Saha Sheila

Table of Contents

CHAPTER ONE

Herbs For Bowel Polyps

Overview

Bowel polyps, additionally referred to as colorectal polyps, are growths that seem to be on the floor of the colon. The colon, or huge gut, is a protracted hole tube at the lowest part of the digestive tract. It's where the frame makes the shop stool.

In most cases, polyps don't cause any signs and are commonly observed on ordinary colon cancer screening exams. However, if you do revel in signs, they will consist of:

Blood inside the stool or rectal bleeding

Pain, diarrhea, or constipation that lasts longer than one week is considered a sign of

Nausea or vomiting when you have a huge polyp

Blood on your bathroom paper or blood-streaked stools can be a demonstration of rectal bleeding and have to be evaluated with the aid of a health practitioner.

Types of bowel polyps

Polyps within the colon can range in length and number. There are 3 varieties of colon polyps:

Hyperplastic polyps are innocent and don't change into most cancers.

Adenomatous polyps are the most common. Although the majority will not develop into most cancers, they do have the potential to develop into colon cancers.

Malignant polyps are polyps that have most cancer cells in them, as determined by a microscopic examination.

What are the reasons for bowel polyps?

Doctors are unable to pinpoint the exact cause of bowel polyps, but polyps are thought to be the result of an abnormal tissue growth.

The frame periodically develops new healthful cells to update antique cells which are broken or now no longer needed. The increase and department of recently formed cells is commonly regulated.

In a few cases, however, new cells develop and divide earlier than they're needed. This extra increase is the reason polyps take shape. The polyps can spread in any location of the colon.

Who is at risk for bowel polyps?

Although the unique reason for bowel polyps isn't known, there are certain elements that may increase your hazard of growing bowel polyps. These hazard elements consist of:

Being over 50.

Being overweight

Having a circle of relatives with a history of polyps or colon cancer

Having polyps in the past

Having ovarian cancer or uterine cancer earlier than age 50

Having an inflammatory situation that impacts the colon, along with crohn's ailment or ulcerative colitis

Having type 2 diabetes that is out of control

Having a hereditary disorder, along with lynch syndrome or gardner's syndrome

Lifestyle behaviors that can contribute to the increase in bowel polyps consist of:

Smokers

Drinking alcohol frequently

Having a sedentary way of life

Eating an excessive-fat food

If you make lifestyle changes to deal with those behaviors, you may be able to reduce your risk of bowelpolyps. Regularly taking a low dose of aspirin and including extra calcium in your food regimen might also assist in saving you from polyps. Other recommendations for lowering your risk may be made by your doctor as well.

CHAPTER TWO

How Are Bowel Polyps Diagnosed?

Polyps may be observed on some exams. These exams may also consist of:

Colonoscopy. During this system, a digital digicam connected to a skinny, bendy tube is threaded via the anus. This permits your health practitioner to view the rectum and colon. If a polyp is observed, your health practitioner can cast off it straight away or take tissue samples for analysis.

Sigmoidoscopy. This screening approach is much like a colonoscopy, but it may be most effectively used to peer into the rectum and decrease the colon. It can't be used to take a biopsy, or a pattern of tissue. If your health practitioner detects a polyp, you'll want to agenda a colonoscopy to have it eliminated.

Barium enema. For this check, your health practitioner injects liquid barium into your rectum, after which he makes use of a unique x-ray to take pics of your colon. Barium makes your colon seem white inside the pictures. Since polyps are dark, they're clean to discover in opposition to the white color.

Ct colonography. This system makes use of a ct test to put together pics of the colon and rectum. After the test, a laptop combines the pics of the colon and rectum to supply each with two 2- and three-d perspectives of the location. A ct colonography is also referred to as a digital colonoscopy on occasion. It can display swollen tissues, masses, ulcers, and polyps.

Stool check. Your health practitioner will come up with a check package and commands for presenting a stool pattern. You'll take the pattern to your health practitioner's workplace for analysis, in particular to check for microscopic bleeding. This check will show when you have blood in your stool, which may be a signal of a polyp.

How are bowel polyps treated?

The best way to deal with bowel polyps is to cast them off. Your health practitioner will probably cast off your polyps throughout a colonoscopy.

The polyps are then tested under the microscope to see what kind of polyp they are and if there are any cancer cells present. Doctors can commonly put off polyps with early-acting surgical treatment.

However, you can want surgical treatment to cast off the polyps if they're huge and can't be eliminated throughout a colonoscopy. In most cases, this may be carried out with the aid of laparoscopic surgical treatment. This kind of surgical treatment is minimally invasive and makes use of a tool known as a laparoscope.

A laparoscope is a protracted, skinny tube with a excessive-depth mild and a excessive-decision digital on the front. The tool is inserted via an incision withinside the abdomen. Once your medical professional has a visible of your colon, they'll cast off the polyps the use of a unique tool.

A pathologist, or a person who focuses on tissue analysis, will take a look at the polyps for cancerous cells.

CHAPTER THREE

How Can Bowel Polyps Be Prevented?

Maintaining a healthy food regimen can assist in saving you from the development of bowel polyps. This consists of consuming extra culmination, veggies, complete grains, and lean meat.

You will also be capable of saving your polyps with the aid of increasing your consumption of vitamin d and calcium. Foods which are wealthy in vitamin d and calcium consist of:

Brussel sprouts

Greek yogurt

Milk

Cheese

Eggs

Liver

Fish

You can also decrease your hazard of bowel polyps with the aid of decreasing your consumption of excessive-fat ingredients, pink meat, and processed ingredients. Quitting smoking and working out often are also essential steps to slow the growth of bowel polyps.

Herbs for bowel polyps

Garlic

Due to its antioxidant properties, garlic can be a useful adjunctive remedy for sufferers with colon cancer. Phytochemicals in garlic consist of allicin and allicin-derived organo-sulfur compounds along with diallyl disulfide may also have very robust houses in decreasing colon polyps with the aid of using blocking off vitamins along with glucose and oxygen.

Green tea

Green tea comes from the leaves of the camellia sinensis plant. It has an inhibitory impact on human colon cancer cellular lines herbal safety however, medical trials have to decide authentic efficacy. Studies propose that epigallocatechin-three-gallate, a lively constituent of inexperienced tea, neutralizes enzymes assisting in the increase of colon polyps. To gain this gain, you ought to drink at least five cups of inexperienced tea every day.

Flax plants

The flax plant is a member of the linaceae family, with the clinical name linum usitatissimum. The seeds are used medicinally. The anti-carcinogenic

properties of flaxseed are attributed to the excessive concentrations of alpha-linolenic acid, an omega-three fatty acid, which seems to guard in opposition to colon cancer, consistent with the south dakota state university.

The flax plant is a member of the linaceae family, with the clinical name linum usitatissimum.

The anti-carcinogenic properties of flaxseed are attributed to the excessive concentrations of alpha-linolenic acid, an omega-three fatty acid, which seems to guard in opposition to colon most cancers, consistent with south dakota state university.

Herbs may also assist in decreasing colon polyps. However, they're now no longer meant to replace traditional cancer remedies. In addition, herbs may also lessen the effectiveness of a few anti-most cancer medications. If you've got most cancers, you have to no longer use herbs without first speaking to your health practitioner.

The colon, or large gut, performs the monumental

task of processing waste within the digestive machine to allow for healthy and clean bowel movements (see reference four).poor bowel movements are symptomatic of a bad colon, which can be attributed to a negative food regimen in addition to environmental toxins. Toxins from meals can be absorbed into the bloodstream rather than removed from within the presence of broken colon walls. Dietary changes can help improve colon fitness and resources for the prevention of digestive issues such as irritable bowel syndrome and colon cancer.

Cruciferous veggies

According to the cancer nutrition centers of america, intake of cruciferous veggies is related to a decreased risk of most cancers, including colon most cancers (see reference five). Cruciferous vegetables incorporate phytonutrients that combat most cancers, especially the sulfur-containing compounds called glucosinolates. Fill your plate with broccoli, cauliflower, bok choy and kale for excellent colon fitness.

CHAPTER FOUR

Starches

Resistant starches are carbs that skip digestion inside the small gut and enter the huge gut in a close-to-authentic shape. These starches promote good bacterial growth in the intestines, which can help with digestive issues, inflammatory bowel disease, and cancer risks. Root veggies along with yams, candy potatoes, and iciness squashes incorporate resistant starches, as do seed hulls, rice, and legumes.

Probiotic-rich foods

Probiotics are beneficial microorganisms that aid in the balance of beneficial to harmful intestinal microflora within the intestines (see reference three).you can assist in restoring negative intestinal fitness with the aid of consuming probiotic-wealthy ingredients such as sauerkraut, miso, yogurt, or kimchi (see reference). According to a study published in the journal of pediatric gastroenterology and nutrition, people with irritable bowel syndrome may benefit from probiotic use.

Supplements and herbs

Vitamin a, glutamine, and fish oil may also assist you in saving money and dealing with irritable bowel disease to enhance colon fitness.

Furthermore, herbs like turmeric have anti-inflammatory properties that may help heal negative intestinal fitness with the aid of decreasing inflammation (see reference 6). The american cancer society cites curcumin, a lively component in turmeric, as having proven anti-most cancerous outcomes in animal laboratory research. Further studies are wanted into its impact on humans.

Other treatments

To date, few herbal treatments or opportunities remedies have been observed to play a giant function in colon cancer prevention. However, preliminary research indicates that the subsequent materials may also help reduce the risk of colon cancer to a small extent. Take a look at some of the key research findings:

Vitamin d

High blood levels of vitamin d can be connected to a decreased hazard of colon cancer, consistent with a study. Analyzing records on 5706 human beings with colorectal most cancers and 7107 healthful individuals, researchers decided that girls with the best tiers of nutrition d had a statistically giant decreased hazard of colon most cancers as compared to people with the bottom tiers. For guys, the hazard has decreased, but now not to a statistically giant degree.

Folate

Making sure you eat sufficient meals reassets of folate (a b vitamin observed in ingredients like spinach, asparagus, and fortified cereals) may also decrease your risk of colon cancer, consistent with a systematic assessment and meta-analysis. However, the studies are blended and extra research is needed. 2ndthe recommended daily consumption of folate is four hundred micrograms (mcg) for adults. Pregnant girls have to eat six hundred mcg every day, at the same time as breastfeeding girls have to eat 500 mcg every day.

Quercetin

In lab exams on cell cultures, scientists have validated that quercetin, an antioxidant observed in tea, may also help stall the increase of colon cancers. What's more, a population-primarily based total study of 2,664 human beings observed that nutritional consumption of quercetin can be connected with a decreased hazard of colon most cancers within the proximal colon (first and center parts). However, this link is no longer observed for colon cancers in the distal colon (remaining part) and is no longer visible in people who already consume a lot of tea. The number five

Quercetin is to be had in complement shape and is additionally evidently observed in ingredients like apples, onions, and berries.

Screening

Screening for colorectal cancer has to start at age forty-five for all adults at common hazard. However, in a few cases, early screening is probably appropriate. People who have a family history of colorectal cancer or colon polyps, as well as those who have an inflammatory bowel disease, should consult with their doctor about their risk and when screening should begin.8th

Because of rising rates of colon cancer diagnoses under the age of 50, the us preventive services task force and the american college of gastroenterology updated their respective medical guidelines for colon cancer screening in spring 2021 to begin at age 45 rather than 50.

A healthy diet

Eating 5 or more servings of culmination and veggies per day, choosing whole grains over processed grains, and limiting processed and red meats can all help to save your colon.

Exercises

For colon cancer prevention, the goal is to do a minimum half-hour of exercise on 5 or extra days of the week. Getting at least 45 minutes of mild or vigorous exercise five or more times per week may also reduce your risk of colon cancer.

The takeaway

Bowel polyps don't commonly reason any signs. They're most customarily observed throughout ordinary colon screenings, along with a colonoscopy or a sigmoidoscopy.

Your best choice for finding out when you have bowel polyps is to have colon screenings often while your health practitioner recommends them. The polyps can regularly be eliminated at the identical time because of the screening system.

Though polyps are commonly benign, doctors most customarily cast them off due to the fact that a few varieties of polyps can later turn into most cancers. Removing bowel polyps can help save your colon from growing.

A healthy food regimen, consisting of ingredients rich in vitamin d, calcium, and fiber, can decrease

your risk of developing
bowel polyps.

THE END

Made in the USA
Middletown, DE
09 February 2022